"AFRICAN BLACK SOAP AIN'T JUST FOR AFRICANS"

A Comprehensive Guide to Using African Black
Soap for Clear, Healthy Skin

Frazier & Cindy Cunningham
Co-Founders of Fra Fra's Naturals

CONTENT

Copyright

INTRODUCTION

CHAPTER ONE

CHAPTER TWO

CHAPTER THREE

CHAPTER FOUR

CHAPTER FIVE

CHAPTER SIX

CHAPTER SEVEN

CHAPTER EIGHT

CHAPTER NINE

CHAPTER TEN

10 SUPER EASY DIY SKINCARE RECIPES YOU CAN MAKE AT HOME

CONCLUSION

FAQ ABOUT FRA FRA'S NATURALS

Copyright

This eBook contains information that has been carefully researched and examined for accuracy. It is intended to help the readers be better informed consumers of skin care products. It is presented as general advice.

This book is not intended to be a substitute for the medical advice of a licensed dermatologist. The reader should consult with their doctor in any matters relating to his/her health. The information provided within this eBook is for general informational purposes only.

While we try to keep the information up-to-date and correct, there are no representations or warranties, express or implied, about the completeness, accuracy, reliability, suitability, or availability with respect to the information, products, services, or related graphics contained in this eBook for any purpose. Any use of this information is at your own risk.

INTRODUCTION

At Fra Fra's Naturals, we believe that natural is better. We not only sell African black soap and shea butter, but we are faithful users as well. Our journey began several years ago when our daughter was diagnosed with eczema. We were desperate to find something that would help her, and we were shocked to learn about the potential side effects of the prescription creams that her doctor was recommending.

We decided to search for a more natural solution, and we quickly discovered the power of African black soap. We were amazed at how well it soothed our daughter's skin and helped to clear up her eczema. We were also impressed by the versatility of African black soap, and we began to use it for ourselves as well.

We now use African black soap for everything from washing our hair to exfoliating our skin. We are so passionate about the benefits of African black soap that we decided to start Fra Fra's Naturals. We want to share our knowledge and experience with others so that they can experience the same amazing results that we have.

This book is a comprehensive guide to African black soap. We will cover everything you need to know, from the history of African black soap to its many uses and benefits. We will also debunk some of the myths and misconceptions about African black soap.

Whether you are new to African black soap or are an experienced user, this book is a must-have for anyone who wants to learn more about this amazing product.

In addition to the informative text, we have also included 10 easy-to-follow DIY skin care recipes that utilize African black soap. These recipes are perfect for people of all skin types, and they are a great way to get started with using African black soap.

We hope that this book will help you to learn more about African black soap and how to use it to improve your skin health. We are confident that you will be amazed at the results.

CHAPTER ONE

WHAT IS AFRICAN BLACK SOAP?

African black soap, also known as *Ango Sopa, Ose Dudu*, or *Alata Simena*, is an all-natural soap that has been used by the people of West Africa for centuries. It is made from the ash of locally harvested plants, such as plantain skins, cocoa pods, and palm kernel shells. African black soap is known for its many benefits, including its ability to cleanse, exfoliate, and moisturize the skin. It is also said to be effective in treating a variety of skin conditions, such as acne, eczema, and psoriasis.

Africa has a rich history of scientific knowledge and innovation. Ancient African cultures had a deep understanding of the natural world, and they developed many ingenious ways to use natural resources. For example, the ancient Egyptians were experts in mathematics, astronomy, and medicine. They also developed a sophisticated system of irrigation, which helped them to create a thriving agricultural civilization.

Unfortunately, the history of African science has been largely ignored by the West. This is due in part to the legacy of colonialism, which sought to portray Africans as primitive and uncivilized. However, there is a growing movement to reclaim the history of African science and to celebrate the contributions that African scientists have made to the world.

The development of African black soap is a testament to the ingenuity and creativity of African people. This soap is a natural, effective, and affordable way to care for the skin. It is also a reminder of the rich history of African science and innovation.

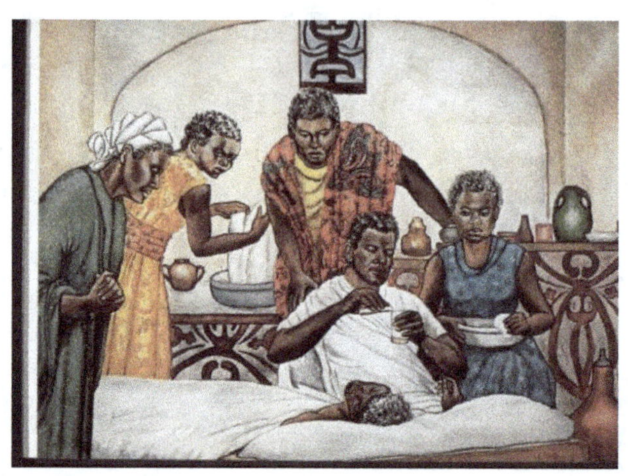

Ancient African civilizations, including those in Egypt, South Africa, and Nigeria, made significant contributions to science and medicine. For example, they developed the use of plants for medicinal purposes, including the use of salicylic acid for pain relief (salicylic acid is the primary ingredient in modern-day aspirin). They also performed medical procedures such as vaccinations, autopsies, brain surgery, and extensive dental work.

This knowledge of plants also gave rise to African black soap, an all-natural cleanser that is made from plant-based ingredients and does not contain preservatives. African black soap is known to be effective in treating a variety of skin conditions, including acne, psoriasis, dermatitis, dark spots, and eczema. It is also naturally infused with vitamins A and E.

African black soap is made with naturally occurring lye from the ashes of the plantain. It is handcrafted by local women in Western Africa, primarily in Ghana. The type of oils used and the exact method of production vary depending on the region. This is why African black soap from different regions may have slight variations in color, consistency, and results.

The popularity of African black soap has led to the production of imitation soaps in the United States and Europe. However, these imitations are often made with artificial ingredients and do not have the same benefits as authentic African black soap. The recipe for authentic African black soap is a closely guarded secret, and the exact ingredients are not known outside of the villages that produce it.

It is important to be aware of the difference between authentic African black soap and imitations when choosing a product for your skin care routine. Authentic African black soap is a natural and effective way to cleanse and moisturize your skin. Imitation soaps may not be as effective and may even cause skin irritation.

CHAPTER TWO

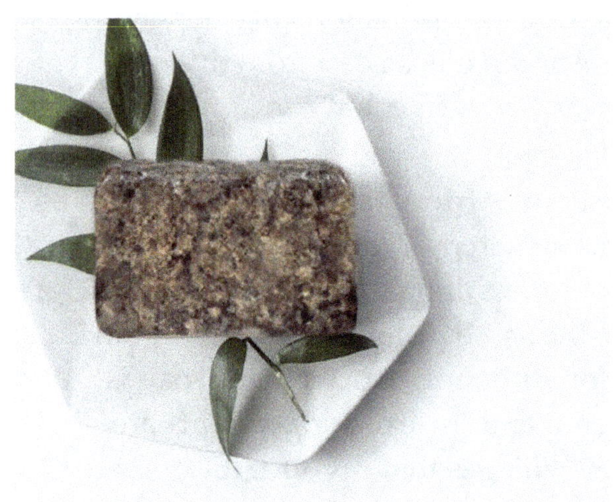

Authentic African black soap is made from simple, organic, plant-based materials that are locally harvested by women. The ingredients are sun-dried and roasted, which gives the soap its deep, rich color. The darker the soap, the more plantain skins it contains. A lighter bar is the result of a higher concentration of cocoa pods.

Plantain

The sun-dried, roasted plantain skins provide a high content of vitamins and minerals, including iron, vitamin A (retinol), vitamin E, and allatonin.

- Vitamin E is a powerful antioxidant that can help to reduce scarring, damage from UV rays, and free radicals. It is also a collagen booster and encourages collagen production.

- Vitamin A, also known as retinol, activates key cells needed to develop tissue that keeps skin firm and healthy. It promotes the production of these cells in the deep layers of skin, resulting in visibly firmer skin.

- Allantoin, which is also found in African shea butter, has a host of benefits:

    o It increases the water content of skin, thus increasing hydration.

    o It naturally exfoliates the outer layer of skin.

    o It kickstarts the healing process by stimulating new tissue growth.

    o It revitalizes skin by promoting cellular regeneration and preventing dryness.

Cocoa pods

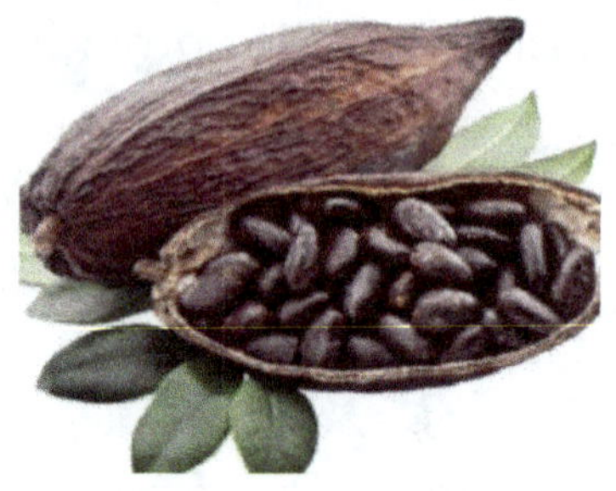

The cocoa pods are rich in antioxidants, including malic acid, procyanidin B1, rosmarinic acid, procyanidin C1, apigenin, and ellagic acid.

- Malic acid is an alpha hydroxy acid that has many benefits for skin and health. It is a humectant, which means it helps the skin to retain moisture and stay hydrated. It is also an anti-inflammatory agent that can reduce swelling, pain, and soreness in muscles. Additionally, it is a pH balancing agent that can brighten and rejuvenate the skin. Finally, it is a gentle exfoliant that can exfoliate the top layer of skin and stimulate ceramide production.

- Procyanidin B1 is a powerful antioxidant that counteracts the harmful effects of free radicals.

- Rosmarinic acid is another powerful antioxidant and anti-inflammatory agent. It has been shown to protect against various forms of cancer, increase circulation, and improve skin tone. It is also antiseptic, which makes it perfect for people with oily or acne-prone skin.

- Apegenin acid has been shown to have multiple benefits. It is an anti-inflammatory, an antioxidant, and a stimulant for blood vessels and hair growth. It is also an anti-irritant, a lightening agent, an anticarcinogen, and an antiseptic.

- Procyanidin C1 acid shares many of the same traits of the other acids, but it also improves the elasticity of skin.

- Ellagic acid is an anticarcinogen, protects against UV damage, brightens skin, fades dark spots, and slows the aging process.

Palm tree leaves and oil

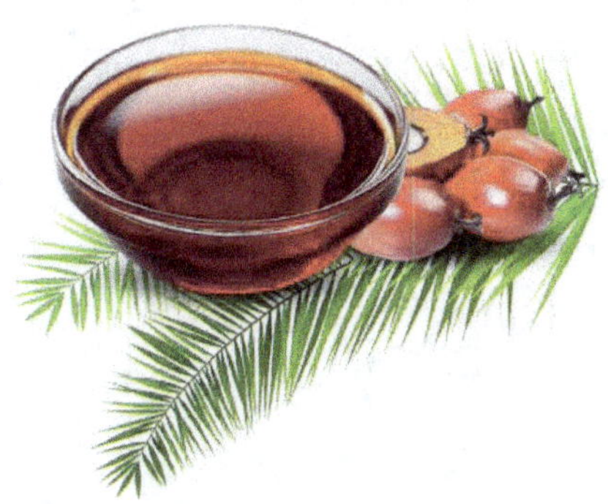

Palm tree leaves and oil are rich in vitamin E (tocotrienol), a form of vitamin E that is more potent than other forms. Tocotrienol is known to promote hair cell growth and prevent hair loss. It is also more effective than other forms of vitamin E at slowing down the aging process and preventing damage to the skin due to free radicals and UV rays. Palm oil is also a refatting agent that restores moisture to hair and skin, leaving the user with softer and more resilient skin.

Shea butter

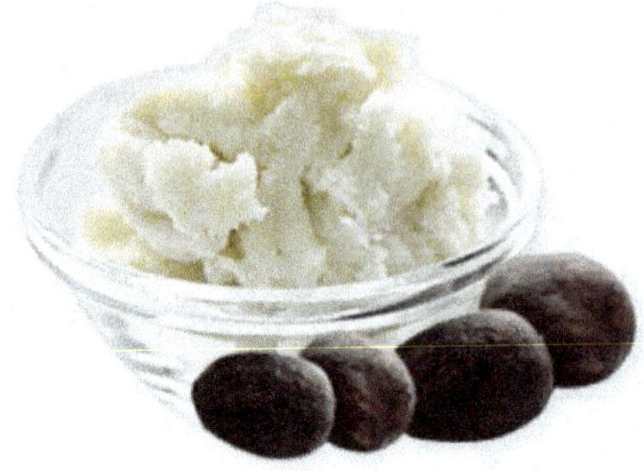

Unrefined shea butter is an excellent source of vitamins A, E, F, and K. It is saturated with fatty acids that moisturize, restore, heal, and protect skin. Shea butter has been shown to be effective in healing burns, scars, dermatitis, psoriasis, and sores, as well as dandruff and stretch marks. It can also diminish wrinkles, brighten skin, and promote cell regeneration.

Overall, African black soap is a natural and effective way to cleanse, exfoliate, and moisturize the skin. It is rich in antioxidants and vitamins that can help to protect the skin from damage and promote healthy skin aging.

CHAPTER THREE

12 POWERFUL BENEFITS OF AFRICAN BLACK SOAP

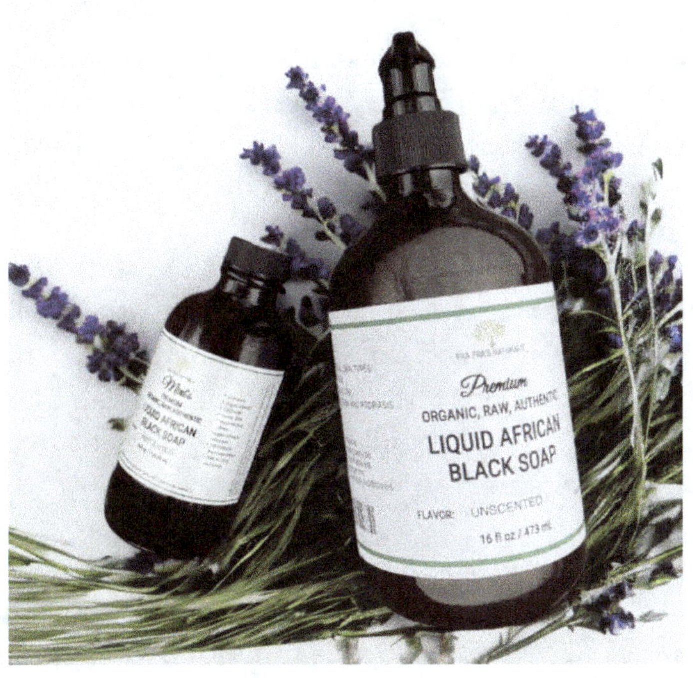

Have you wondered what all the hype is surrounding African black soap? Do you want to know if it lives up to its reputation? If so let me assure you that yes, it does everything that heard and probably more.

The all-natural ingredients are beneficial individually but when combined they create a powerful cleanser.

An all-natural daily cleanser: African black soap is made from all-natural ingredients, including plantain skins, cocoa pods, palm oil, and shea butter. These ingredients are known for their cleansing, moisturizing, and exfoliating properties. African black soap produces a rich lather that gently removes dirt, oil, dead cells, and other impurities from the skin. It is also non-drying, so it is gentle on even the most sensitive skin.

Good for all skin types: African black soap is suitable for all skin types, including oily, dry, and sensitive skin. The shea butter in African black soap helps to moisturize dry skin, while the plantain skins and cocoa pods help to exfoliate and remove dead skin cells.

Natural exfoliator: African black soap is a gentle exfoliator that helps to remove dead skin cells and reveal new, healthy skin. The plantain skins and cocoa pods in African black soap contain natural exfoliants that help to slough away dead skin cells without irritating the skin.

Soothes and heals eczema: African black soap has anti-inflammatory and moisturizing properties that can help to soothe and heal eczema. The shea butter in African black soap helps to hydrate the skin and reduce inflammation, while the plantain skins and cocoa pods help to remove dead skin cells and promote healing.

Reduces hyperpigmentation and dark spots: African black soap contains vitamin A, which is known to help reduce hyperpigmentation and dark spots. The shea butter in African black soap also helps to moisturize the skin and protect it from sun damage, which can help to reduce the appearance of hyperpigmentation and dark spots.

Good for acne-prone skin: African black soap has antibacterial and anti-inflammatory properties that can help to treat acne. The shea butter in African black soap helps to moisturize the skin and reduce inflammation, while the plantain skins and cocoa pods help to remove excess oil and dirt from the skin, which can help to prevent acne breakouts.

Calms psoriasis: African black soap contains natural ingredients that can help to calm psoriasis, including shea butter, plantain skins, and cocoa pods. The shea butter in African black soap helps to moisturize the skin and reduce inflammation, while the plantain skins and cocoa pods help to remove dead skin cells and promote healing.

Antimicrobial and antifungal properties: African black soap has antimicrobial and antifungal properties that can help to fight bacteria and fungi that can cause skin infections. The shea butter in African black soap helps to create a barrier on the skin that can help to prevent the growth of bacteria and fungi.

Minimizes wrinkles: African black soap contains antioxidants that can help to protect the skin from damage caused by free radicals. Free radicals are unstable molecules that can damage cells and contribute to the signs of aging. The antioxidants in African black soap can help to neutralize free radicals and protect the skin from damage.

Alleviates razor bumps: African black soap can help to alleviate razor bumps by moisturizing the skin and preventing ingrown hairs. The shea butter in African black soap helps to soften the skin and protect it from irritation, while the plantain skins and cocoa pods help to remove dead skin cells and promote healing.

Dandruff treatment: African black soap can help to treat dandruff by removing excess oil and dirt from the scalp, which can help to prevent dandruff flakes. The shea butter in African black soap also helps to moisturize the scalp and relieve dryness.

Makeup remover: African black soap can be used to remove makeup without stripping the skin of its natural oils. The shea butter in African black soap helps to moisturize the skin, while the plantain skins and cocoa pods help to remove makeup and impurities.

Overall, African black soap is a versatile and effective natural cleanser that can be used to treat a variety of skin problems. It is gentle enough for all skin types and is made from all-natural ingredients. If you are looking for a natural way to improve the appearance of your skin, African black soap is a great option.

CHAPTER FOUR

HOW TO USE AFRICAN BLACK SOAP

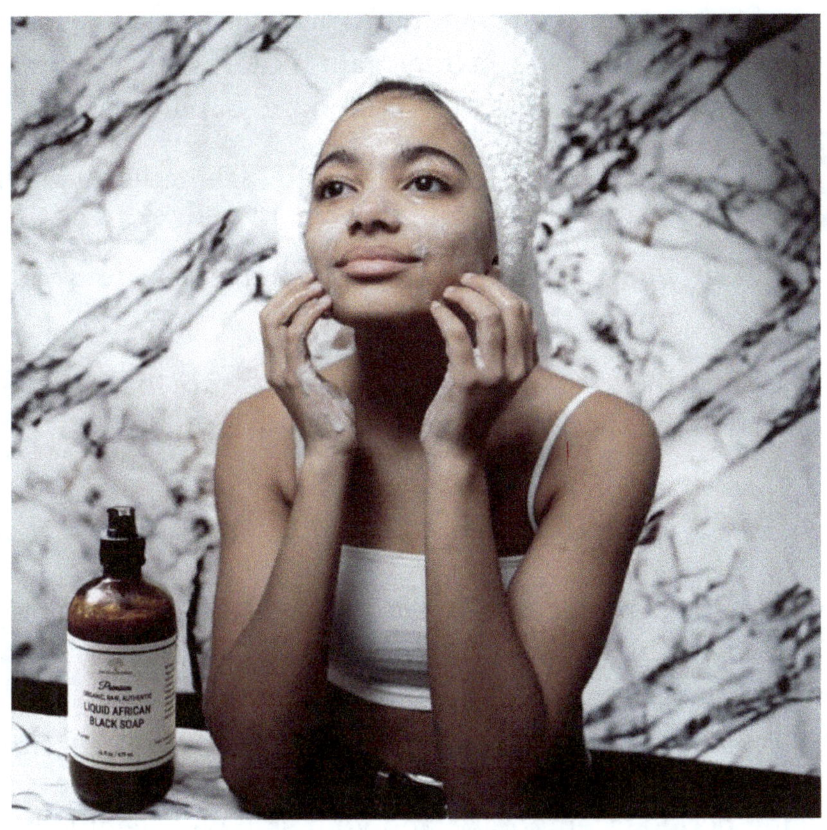

African black soap is a natural, all-purpose soap that can be used for a variety of skin care needs. However, it is important to follow some guidelines when using it for the first time.

- Start with a small amount. African black soap is very concentrated, so it is important to start with a small amount. You can always add more soap if needed.

- Wet your skin before applying the soap. This will help to prevent the soap from drying out your skin.

- Gently massage the soap into your skin. Do not scrub your skin, as this can irritate it.

- Rinse the soap off thoroughly. Make sure to rinse away all of the soap, as residue can clog your pores.

Purge Period

Some people experience a purging period when they first start using African black soap. This is a normal process that happens as the soap removes impurities from the skin. The purging period can last for a few weeks, and during this time, you may experience breakouts or dryness. However, the purging period is temporary, and your skin will eventually clear up.

Burning Sensation

Some people also experience a burning sensation when they first start using African black soap. This is usually due to the soap's high pH level. The burning sensation should subside after a few uses. If it does not, you may be allergic to one of the ingredients in the soap.

Allergies

African black soap is made from natural ingredients, but it is still possible to be allergic to one of the ingredients. If you experience any allergic reaction, such as redness, itching, or swelling, discontinue use of the soap and consult with a doctor or dermatologist.

Overall, African black soap is a safe and effective soap for most people. However, it is important to follow the guidelines above when using it for the first time.

Do a skin test first!

Always do a patch test before using African black soap for the first time. This is especially important if you have sensitive skin or allergies. To do a patch test, apply a small amount of soap to the inside of your wrist or elbow. Wait 24 hours to see if you have any reaction. If you do, such as redness, itching, or swelling, do not use the soap.

A slight burning or stinging sensation is normal when first using African black soap. This is because the soap is working to remove impurities from your skin. The burning sensation should subside after a few uses.

If you experience any other side effects, such as severe burning, itching, or swelling, stop using the soap and see a doctor or dermatologist. You may be allergic to one of the ingredients in the soap.

Do not apply directly to the face!

When switching to African black soap, it is best to start by not applying it directly to your skin. Instead, use a soft washcloth or bath sponge to lather the soap. If you are using your hands, break off a small piece of soap and roll it into a small ball to remove any sharp plant residue. Lather up lightly at first to avoid the feeling of burning or overly tight skin. Rinse with warm, not hot, water and pat dry. Immediately follow up with a moisturizer. Shea butter is a great choice, as it is both organic and all-natural, and it has amazing skin benefits. It is also a native product of the same region that produces African black soap.

Do not use as a daily facial wash initially!

African black soap is a natural, all-purpose soap that can be used for a variety of skin care needs, including the face. However, it is important to start slowly and gradually introduce it to your face, as it can be harsh for some people.

- Start by using it once or twice a week. This will give your skin time to adjust to the soap and prevent any irritation.

- Wet your face before applying the soap. This will help to prevent the soap from drying out your skin.

- Gently massage the soap into your face. Do not scrub your face, as this can irritate it.

- Rinse the soap off thoroughly. Make sure to rinse away all of the soap, as residue can clog your pores.

If you have sensitive skin, you may want to start with even less frequent use, such as once a week. You can also try diluting the soap with water before applying it to your face.

Be sure to take care around the eyes and nose. The skin in these areas is thinner and more delicate, so be extra gentle when applying the soap.

Over time, you may be able to increase the frequency of use. However, it is important to listen to your skin and stop using the soap if it causes any irritation.

Do not over exfoliate!

African black soap is a natural, all-purpose soap that is gentler on the skin than traditional soap. However, it is still important to use it gently, especially when you are first starting out.

Here are some tips for using African black soap gently:

- Do not use a loofah, mitt, or facial brush. These tools can irritate your skin and make it more prone to breakouts.

- Gently massage the soap into your skin. Do not scrub.

- Rinse the soap off thoroughly. Make sure to rinse away all of the soap, as residue can clog your pores.

If you have sensitive skin, you may want to start by using African black soap once a week and gradually increase the frequency of use as your skin adjusts. You can also try diluting the soap with water before applying it to your skin.

It is okay to use African black soap with other ingredients for additional exfoliation but be sure to use a gentle circular motion. Some good ingredients to use include sugar, salt, or oatmeal.

After the initial purging and transition period, you may find that you can use African black soap more often without irritation. However, it is always important to listen to your skin and stop using the soap if it causes any problems.

Always follow up with a good moisturizer. African black soap can be drying, so it is important to moisturize your skin after using it.

Here are some additional tips for using African black soap gently:

- Look for a soap that is specifically formulated for sensitive skin.

- Test the soap on a small area of your skin before using it all over.

- If you have any concerns, talk to your doctor or dermatologist.

Here are some additional things to keep in mind when using African black soap:

- African black soap has a pH level of 7 to 8, which is similar to the pH level of the skin. This makes it less likely to irritate the skin than traditional soap, which has a pH level of 9 to 10.

- African black soap is a natural exfoliant, which means it can help to remove dead skin cells and promote cell turnover. However, it is important to use it gently, as too much exfoliation can irritate the skin.

- African black soap can be used to treat a variety of skin conditions, including acne, eczema, and psoriasis. However, it is important to talk to your doctor or dermatologist before using it for any medical condition.

CHAPTER FIVE

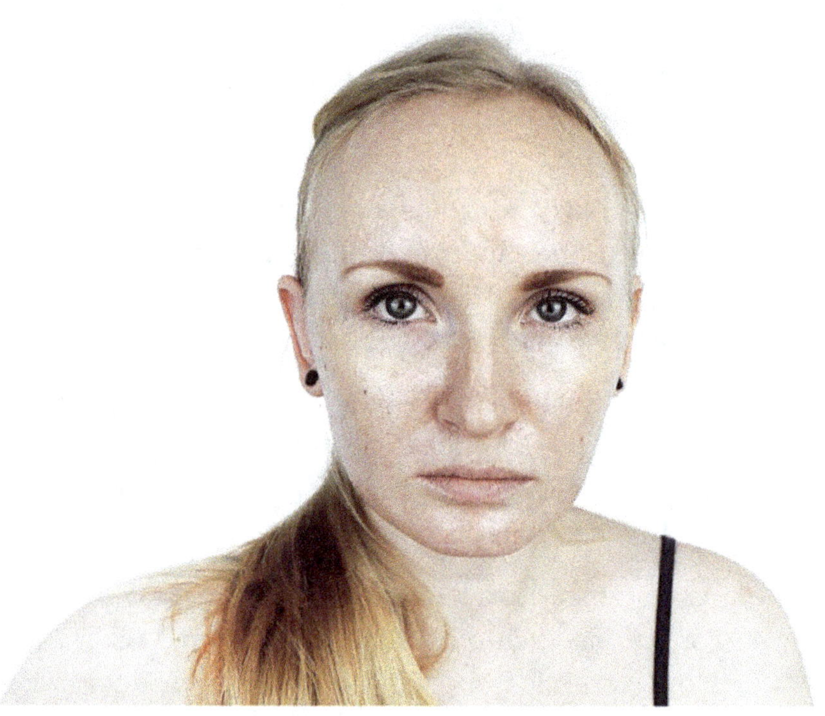

Oily skin is a common skin type that occurs when the sebaceous glands in the skin produce too much sebum, an oily substance that helps to keep the skin moist. While oily skin can be frustrating to deal with, it does have some advantages. For example, oily skin is less likely to wrinkle prematurely than other skin types.

There are a number of things that can cause oily skin, including genetics, hormones, diet, stress, and certain medications. If you have oily skin, it is important to cleanse your skin daily with a gentle cleanser that will not strip away the skin's natural oils. African black soap is a good option for oily skin because it is a natural cleanser that does not contain harsh chemicals.

When you first start using African black soap, your skin may feel tight and dry for a few weeks. This is because the soap is removing excess oil from your skin. However, after this initial purging period, your skin should start to feel less oily and more balanced.

It is important to moisturize your skin after using African black soap to prevent it from drying out. Look for a moisturizer that is non-comedogenic, which means it will not clog your pores. Some good options for oily skin include unrefined shea butter, jojoba oil, or rosehip oil.

Here are some additional tips for caring for oily skin:

- Avoid using harsh cleansers or scrubs.

- Use a toner to remove excess oil and dirt from your skin.

- Moisturize your skin regularly with a non-comedogenic moisturizer.

- Avoid touching your face throughout the day.

- Wash your face twice a day.

- Use sunscreen every day, even if it is cloudy.

CHAPTER SIX

AFRICAN BLACK SOAP FORSENSITIVE/ REACTIVE SKIN

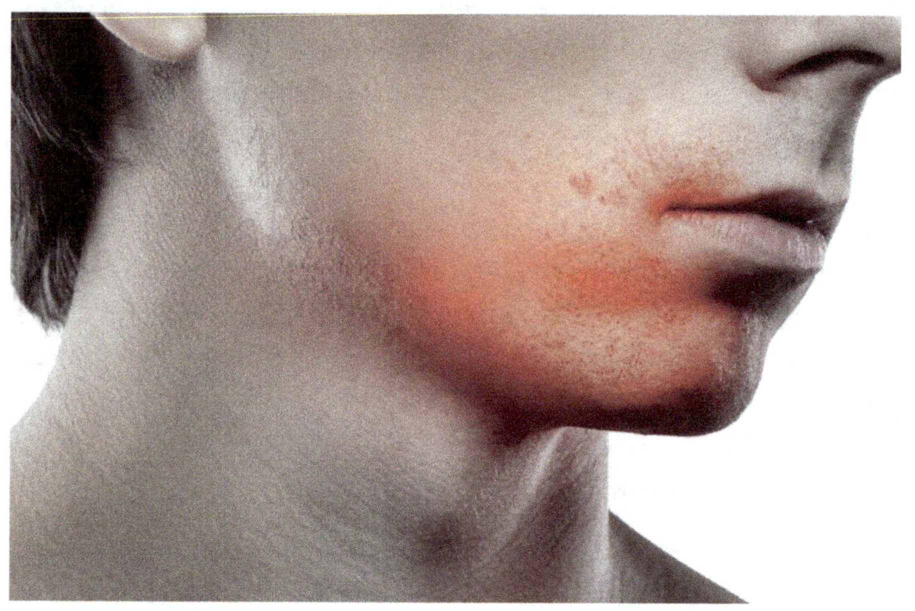

Sensitive skin is a skin type that is easily irritated by certain products or environmental factors. It can be caused by a variety of things, including genetics, allergies, and environmental factors.

People with sensitive skin may experience the following symptoms:

- Dryness

- Irritation

- Burning

- Stinging

- Redness

- Rashes

- Acne

If you have sensitive skin, it is important to avoid using products that contain harsh chemicals, fragrances, or dyes. African black soap is a good option for sensitive skin because it is a natural soap that does not contain these ingredients.

How to Use African Black Soap on Sensitive Skin

Here are some tips for using African black soap on sensitive skin:

1. Do a patch test before using the soap on a larger area of your skin. Apply a small amount of the soap to a patch of skin on your inner wrist. If there is no reaction after 24 hours, you can start using the soap on a small area of your body, such as your back.

2. Start by using the soap once a week and gradually increase the frequency of use as your skin adjusts.

3. Be gentle when washing your skin. Do not scrub.

4. Rinse the soap off thoroughly.

5. Always follow up with a moisturizer.

If you experience any irritation or redness while using African black soap, discontinue use.

CHAPTER SEVEN

AFRICAN BLACK SOAP FOR DRYSKIN

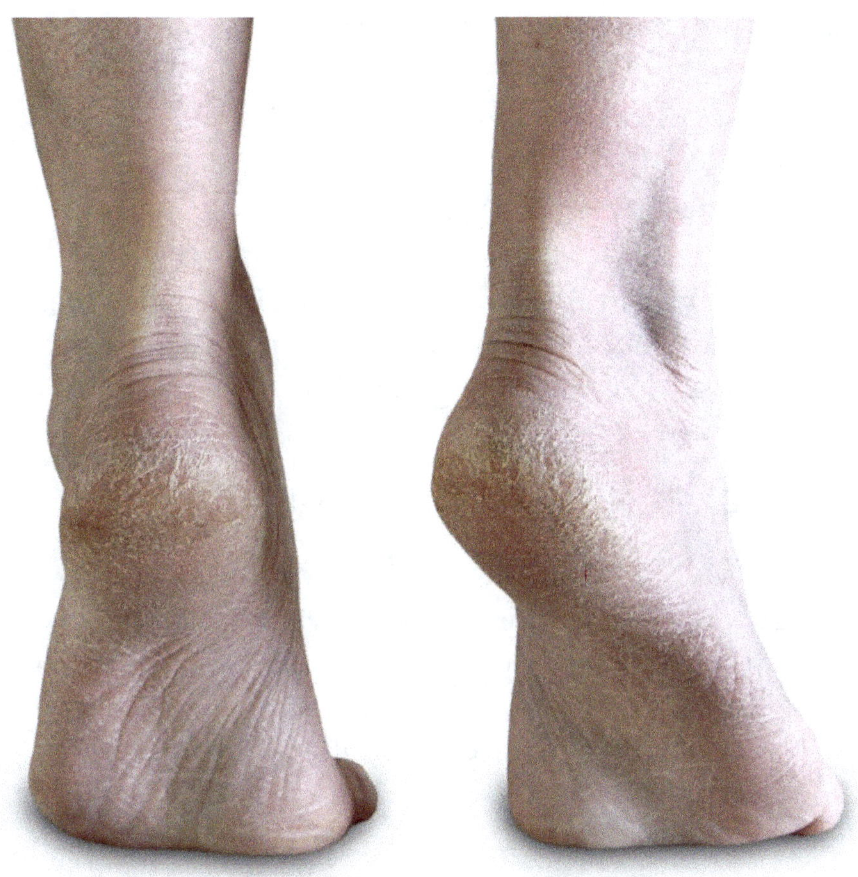

Dry skin is a common skin type that occurs when the skin does not produce enough natural oils. This can lead to a number of problems, including itchiness, flakiness, and premature aging.

There are a number of things that can cause dry skin, including genetics, climate, and certain medical conditions. If you have dry skin, it is important to use a gentle cleanser that will not strip away the skin's natural oils. African black soap is a good option for dry skin because it is a natural cleanser that does not contain harsh chemicals.

How to Use African Black Soap on Dry Skin

Here are some tips for using African black soap on dry skin:

1. Start by using the soap once a week in a limited area, such as your inner wrist. If there is no reaction after 24 hours, you can start using the soap on a larger area of your body.

2. Be gentle when washing your skin. Do not scrub.

3. Rinse the soap off thoroughly.

4. Always follow up with a moisturizer. Look for a moisturizer that is non-comedogenic, which means it will not clog your pores. Some good options for dry skin include unrefined shea butter, jojoba oil, or rosehip oil.

Here are some other tips for caring for dry skin:

- Avoid hot water and harsh soaps.

- Use a humidifier in your home.

- Take cool baths or showers.

- Apply moisturizer to your skin throughout the day.

- Avoid scratching your skin.

By following these tips, you can help to keep your dry skin hydrated and comfortable.

CHAPTER EIGHT

AFRICAN BLACK SOAP FOR SKIN CONDITIONS

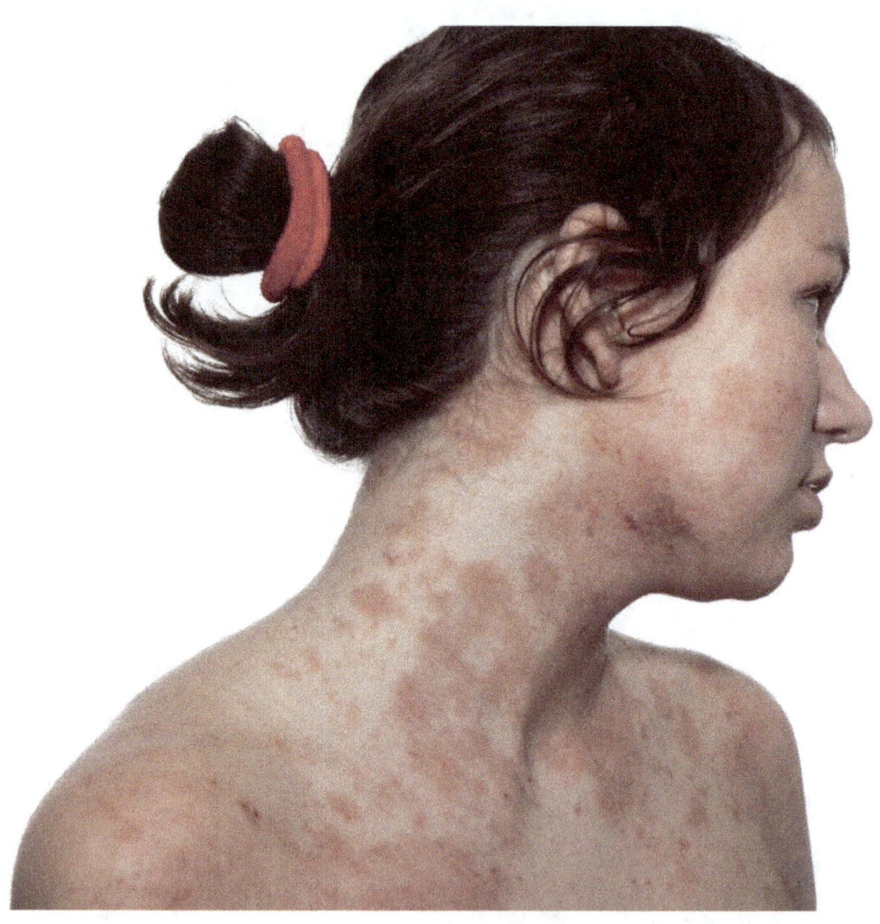

African black soap is a natural soap made from shea butter, palm oil, and plantain ash. It has been used for centuries to treat a variety of skin conditions, including:

- Rosacea: A chronic skin condition that causes redness, flushing, and pimples on the face.

- Eczema: A skin condition that causes inflammation, itching, and rashes.

- Dermatitis: A general term for skin inflammation.

- Psoriasis: A skin condition that causes red, scaly patches.

- Rashes: A general term for skin irritation that can be caused by a variety of factors, such as allergies, infections, or medications.

- Fungal infections: A type of infection caused by fungi.

- Burns: A type of injury caused by heat, cold, chemicals, or radiation.

African black soap is effective for these skin conditions because it has a number of beneficial properties, including:

- Anti-inflammatory: African black soap helps to reduce inflammation, which is a major underlying factor in many skin conditions.

- Antibacterial: African black soap helps to kill bacteria, which can help to prevent infection.

- Exfoliating: African black soap helps to remove dead skin cells, which can help to improve the appearance of the skin.

- Moisturizing: African black soap contains shea butter, which is a natural moisturizer that helps to keep the skin hydrated.

If you are considering using African black soap to treat a skin condition, it is important to talk to your doctor or dermatologist first. They can help you determine if African black soap is right for you and can advise you on how to use it safely.

Here are some additional tips for using African black soap for skin conditions:

- Start by using the soap once a day and gradually increase the frequency as tolerated.

- Be gentle when washing your skin. Do not scrub.

- Rinse the soap off thoroughly.

- Follow up with a moisturizer, especially if your skin is dry.

If you experience any irritation or redness while using African black soap, discontinue use.

CHAPTER NINE

WHY AND HOW TO BUY AUTHENTIC RAW UNREFINED AFRICAN BLACK SOAP

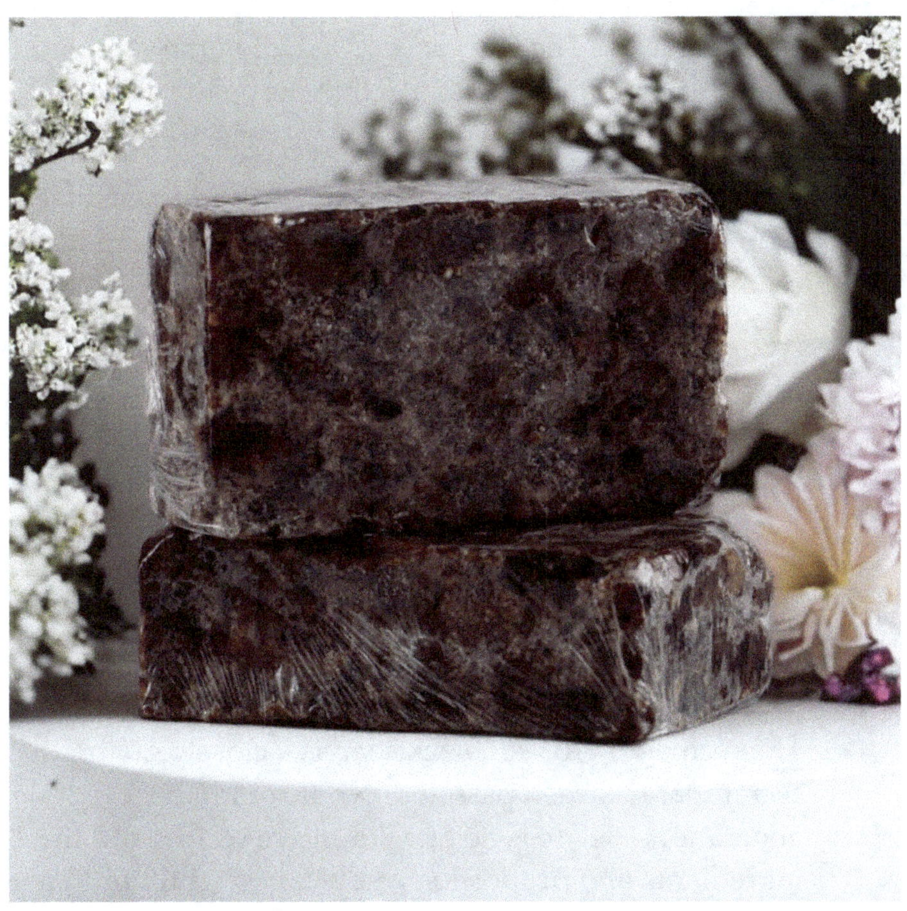

Buying authentic African black soap can be confusing, as there are many imitations on the market. These imitations may not have the same healing properties as authentic

African black soap, and they may also contain harmful chemicals.

Here are some tips for buying authentic African black soap:

- Buy from a reputable seller: Look for a seller that has a good reputation and that sells authentic African black soap.

- Read the label: The label should list all of the ingredients, and it should say that the soap is made with shea butter, palm oil, and plantain ash.

- Look for the color and texture: Authentic African black soap is typically dark brown or black in color and has a crumbly texture.

- Avoid soaps that are too smooth or have a strong fragrance: These soaps are likely to be imitations.

If you are still unsure whether or not a soap is authentic, you can contact the seller and ask them for more information.

Here are some additional things to keep in mind when buying African black soap:

- The recipe for African black soap is a closely guarded secret that has been passed down through the generations. There is no one definitive recipe, and the ingredients and proportions may vary slightly from region to region.

- African black soap is typically made in small batches using traditional methods. This makes it more

expensive than mass-produced soaps, but it also
ensures that the soap is of high quality.

- African black soap is a natural product, and it may not
  be suitable for everyone. If you have sensitive skin, it is
  best to patch test the soap on a small area of your skin
  before using it on a larger area.

Why should I care if it is authentic or not?

African black soap is a natural soap made from shea butter,
palm oil, and plantain ash. It has been used for centuries to
cleanse and protect the skin. However, there is a growing
market for fake African black soap, which is often made with
cheap ingredients and chemicals.

Here are some key differences between authentic and fake
African black soap:

- Color: Authentic African black soap is not jet black. It is
  typically a variation of dark brown to light brown. Any
  African black soap that is jet black in color is not
  authentic.

- Texture: Authentic African black soap is not smooth. It
  is made from natural ingredients and is often chunky
  and has some ash particles in it. If you find a bar of
  African black soap that is smooth to the touch and has
  a uniform shape, it is fake.

- Hardness: Authentic African black soap is soft. This is
  due to its high natural glycerin content. Fake African

black soap is often hard because it is made with cheap ingredients that do not contain glycerin.

- Scent: Authentic African black soap has a natural, earthy smell. Fake African black soap often has a strong fragrance, which is added to mask the smell of the cheap ingredients.

Guidelines for Buying African Black Soap

To avoid buying fake African black soap, follow these guidelines:

- Buy African black soap from a trusted vendor.

- Make sure the label lists all-natural ingredients.

- Look for African black soap that is labeled as raw and unrefined.

- Avoid African black soap that has added fragrances.

- If you are buying liquid African black soap, make sure it is labeled as unrefined and contains essential oils.

By following these guidelines, you can be sure to buy authentic African black soap that will benefit your skin.

CHAPTER TEN

HOW TO STORE AFRICAN BLACK SOAP

When you purchase your first bar of African black soap, you will notice that it is different from traditional soap. Authentic African black soap is brown, not black, and it is not uniform in shape, size, or color. It is also very soft and has a high natural glycerin content. This means that it can draw moisture from the air, which is good for your skin. However, it also means that it can soften quickly if left out in the bathroom.

To prevent your African black soap from softening too quickly, store it in a dry container or an airtight plastic bag. You can also leave it in the soap holder but be sure to drain it first. African black soap does not go bad, so you can store it for a long time if it is stored properly.

The Dangers of Toxic Skin Care Products

Our skin is our body's largest organ and it protects us from the elements. It also helps to regulate our body temperature and remove toxins. However, many of the skin care products that we use are loaded with chemicals that can be harmful to our health.

The average person uses 10 different skin care products daily. While this may not seem like a lot, it adds up over time. And many of these products contain chemicals that can be absorbed into our skin and bloodstream.

Some of the most common harmful chemicals found in skin care products include:

- Parabens: These chemicals are used as preservatives in many skin care products. They have been linked to cancer and reproductive problems.

- Phthalates: These chemicals are used to make plastics soft and flexible. They have been linked to reproductive problems and developmental disorders.

- Formaldehyde: This chemical is used as a disinfectant in some skin care products. It can cause allergic reactions and respiratory problems.

- Fragrance: Many skin care products contain artificial fragrances, which can be made up of hundreds of chemicals, some of which are known to be harmful.

- Triclosan: This is an antibacterial agent that has been linked to antibiotic resistance.

- Sulfates: These are detergents that can irritate our skin and eyes.

The long-term effects of exposure to these chemicals are not fully known. However, some studies have shown that they can contribute to increased chances of birth defects, sperm damage, infertility, and some cancers.

The good news is that there are many natural and safe skin care products available. These products are made with plant-based ingredients and are free of harmful chemicals. When choosing skin care products, it is important to read the labels carefully and look for products that are labeled as "natural" or "organic."

If you are concerned about the health risks of toxic skin care products, there are a few things you can do:

- Read the labels carefully and avoid products that contain harmful chemicals.

- Look for products that are labeled as "natural" or "organic."

- Choose products that are made with plant-based ingredients.

- Ask your doctor or dermatologist for recommendations for safe skin care products.

By taking these steps, you can protect your health and your skin from the harmful effects of toxic skin care products.

Here are some additional tips for choosing safe skin care products:

- Look for products that are fragrance-free.

- Avoid products that contain artificial colors.

- Choose products that are hypoallergenic.

- Test new products on a small area of your skin before using them on a larger area.

*Note: All of these recipes require organic liquid or softened African black soap. To soften African black soap, you can grate a small piece of soap with a cheese grater and add it to a small pot. Spray the shavings with a small amount of water and heat the pot on low heat. Stir the mixture and add more water as needed until it reaches the consistency of Vaseline.

You can buy organic raw unrefined African black soap from a variety of retailers, including frafrasnaturals.com.

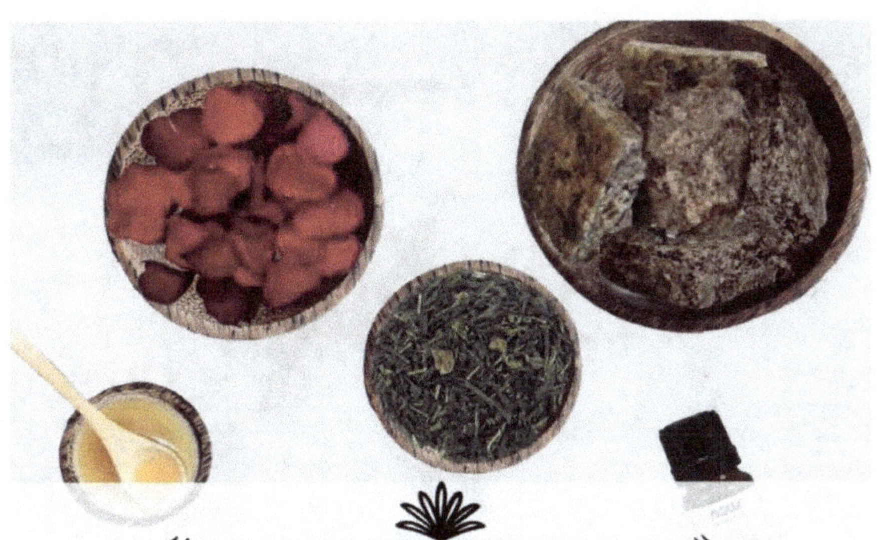

10 Super Easy DIY African Black Soap Skin Care Recipes You Can Do At Home

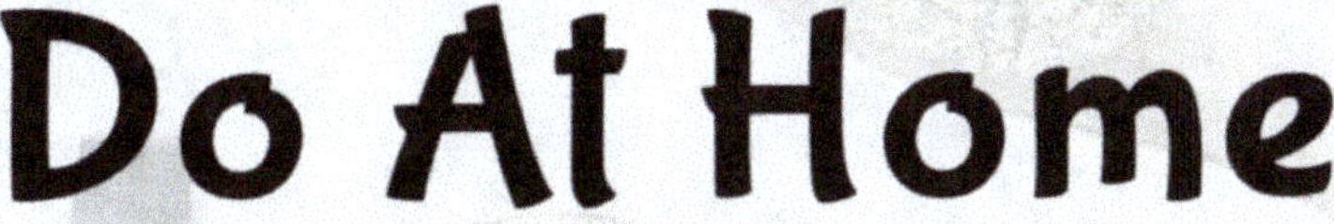

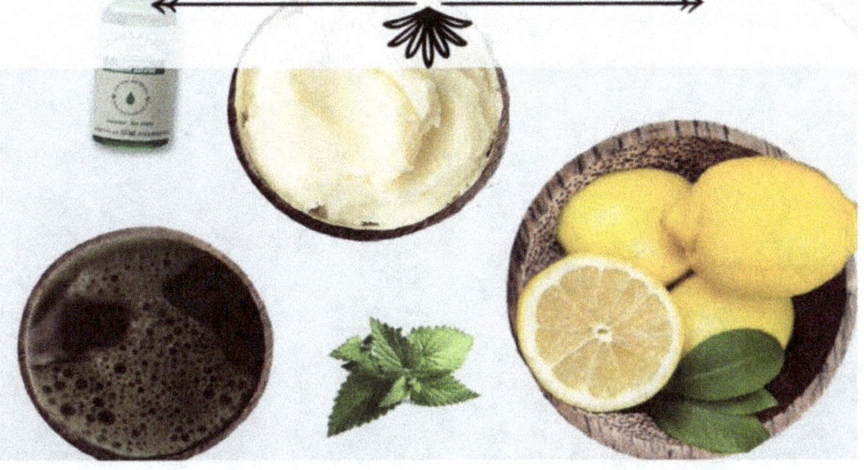

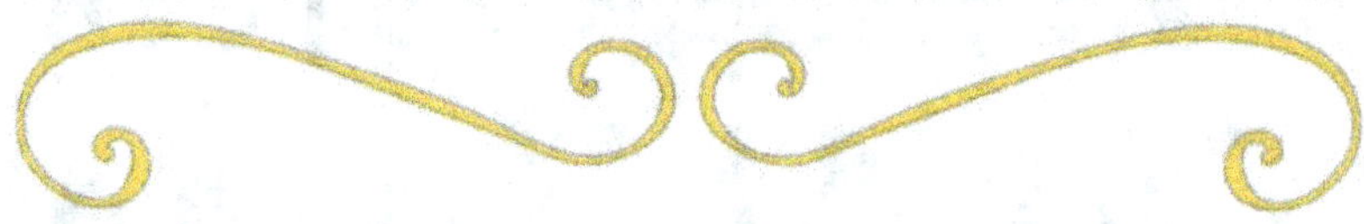

REVITALIZING AFRICAN BLACK SOAP
& LEMON SUGAR BODY SCRUB

African black soap is a natural skin care powerhouse that cleanses, exfoliates, and evens out skin tones. The addition of lemon juice, honey, and apple cider vinegar brightens and hydrates the skin. This gentle scrub helps control breakouts, excess oil, and detoxifies the skin, leaving it feeling refreshed.

Ingredients:

- 2 cups organic sugar
- ¼ cup organic coconut oil
- 1 tablespoon organic lemon juice
- ½ tablespoon raw organic honey
- 1 teaspoon apple cider vinegar
- 2 tablespoons liquid or softened African black soap

Instructions:

1. Pour the sugar into a jar or container.
2. Add the coconut oil and lemon juice and mix until well combined.
3. Stir in the honey, apple cider vinegar, and African black soap until a smooth paste forms.
4. Apply the scrub to your damp skin in a gentle, circular motion.
5. Rinse the scrub off with warm water.

Tips:

- Use this scrub 2-3 times per week for best results.

- Store the scrub in an airtight container in a cool, dark place.

- If you have sensitive skin, you may want to start with a smaller amount of the scrub and gradually increase the amount as your skin gets used to it.

Warnings:

- Avoid using this scrub on open wounds or irritated skin.

- If you experience any redness, itching, or irritation, discontinue use.

AFRICAN BLACK
SOAP ALMOND &
VANILLA BODY
SCRUB

This body scrub will leave your skin feeling soft, nourished, and hydrated. The African black soap, almond and vanilla essential oils work to penetrate deep within the skin, leaving you with baby-smooth skin from head to toe.

Ingredients:

- ½ cup organic sugar

- ½ cup organic oats

- 2 teaspoons almond essential oil

- 2 teaspoons vanilla essential oil

- 2 tablespoons liquid or softened African black soap

Instructions:

1. In a jar or container, combine the sugar and oats.

2. Add the essential oils and African black soap.

3. Mix until well combined.

4. Apply the scrub to your damp skin in a gentle, circular motion.

5. Rinse the scrub off with warm water.

Tips:

- Use this scrub 2-3 times per week for best results.

- Store the scrub in an airtight container in a cool, dark place.

- If you have sensitive skin, you may want to start with a smaller amount of the scrub and gradually increase the amount as your skin gets used to it.

Warnings:

- Avoid using this scrub on open wounds or irritated skin.

- If you experience any redness, itching, or irritation, discontinue use.

Here are some additional benefits of the ingredients used in this scrub:

- Organic sugar is a natural exfoliant that helps to remove dead skin cells and reveal smooth, new skin.

- Organic oats are rich in antioxidants and vitamins that help to nourish and protect the skin.

- Almond essential oil is known for its moisturizing and skin-soothing properties.

- Vanilla essential oil has a calming and relaxing scent that can help to reduce stress and anxiety.

This scrub is a great way to pamper yourself and give your skin the TLC it deserves. So why not give it a try today?

AFRICAN BLACK SOAP &

ROSE BODY SCRUB

Rose petals are a natural cleanser that can help to reduce the appearance of acne, release antioxidants, and tone the skin. When mixed with moisturizing coconut and almond oil, this scrub can leave your skin feeling soft, smooth, and radiant.

Ingredients:

- ¾ cup organic unrefined shea butter
- ½ cup rose petals
- ½ cup organic sugar
- 2 teaspoons almond essential oil
- 2 tablespoons organic liquid or softened African black soap

Instructions:

1. In a jar or container, combine the shea butter and rose petals.
2. Add the sugar and almond essential oil.
3. Mix until well combined.
4. Let the scrub sit for at least 30 minutes to allow the oils to soak into the petals.
5. Apply the scrub to your damp skin in a gentle, circular motion.
6. Rinse the scrub off with warm water.

Tips:

- Use this scrub 2-3 times per week for best results.

- Store the scrub in an airtight container in a cool, dark place.

- If you have sensitive skin, you may want to start with a smaller amount of the scrub and gradually increase the amount as your skin gets used to it.

Warnings:

- Avoid using this scrub on open wounds or irritated skin.

- If you experience any redness, itching, or irritation, discontinue use.

Here are some additional benefits of the ingredients used in this scrub:

- Shea butter is a natural moisturizer that helps to keep the skin hydrated and soft.

- Rose petals are a natural astringent that helps to tighten the pores and reduce the appearance of acne.

- Sugar is a natural exfoliant that helps to remove dead skin cells and reveal smooth, new skin.

- Almond essential oil is a natural antiseptic that helps to fight bacteria and infection.

- African black soap is a natural cleanser that helps to detoxify the skin and remove impurities.

This scrub is made with natural ingredients that are gentle on your skin. It will leave you feeling clean, smooth, and refreshed.

ENERGIZING AFRICAN BLACK SOAP & GREEN TEA SCRUB

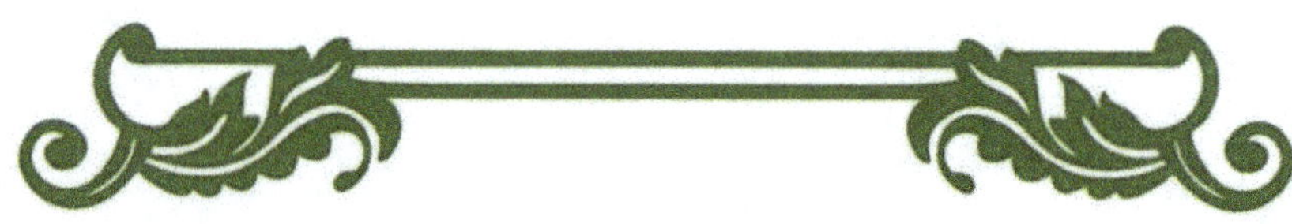

This refreshing DIY scrub is perfect for a day of self-care. It is full of antioxidants and amino acids to help "wake up" your skin.

Ingredients:

- 1 cup organic sugar
- 1 tablespoon organic liquid or softened African black soap*
- 1 organic green tea bag
- 3 tablespoons organic unrefined shea butter
- 1 tablespoon raw organic honey
- 1 teaspoon lavender essential oil (optional)

Instructions:

1. In a bowl, combine the sugar, African black soap, and green tea bag.
2. Steep the green tea bag in hot water for 3-5 minutes, then remove the bag and squeeze out any excess liquid.
3. Add the shea butter, honey, and essential oil (if using).
4. Mix until well combined.
5. Apply the scrub to your damp skin in a gentle, circular motion.
6. Rinse thoroughly with warm water.

Tips:

- This scrub can be stored in an airtight container in the refrigerator for up to 2 weeks.

- If you have sensitive skin, you may want to start with a smaller amount of the scrub and gradually increase the amount as your skin gets used to it.

- Avoid using this scrub on open wounds or irritated skin.

Here are some of the benefits of the ingredients used in this scrub:

- Sugar is a natural exfoliant that helps to remove dead skin cells and reveal smooth, new skin.

- African black soap is a natural cleanser that helps to detoxify the skin and remove impurities.

- Green tea is a natural antioxidant that helps to protect the skin from damage.

- Shea butter is a natural moisturizer that helps to keep the skin hydrated and soft.

- Honey is a natural humectant that helps to draw moisture into the skin.

- Lavender essential oil is a natural calming agent that can help to reduce stress and anxiety.

This scrub is full of antioxidants and amino acids to help 'wake up' your skin. Try it today and see the difference!

ULTRA RELAXING CHAMOMILE & AFRICAN BLACK SOAP SCRUB

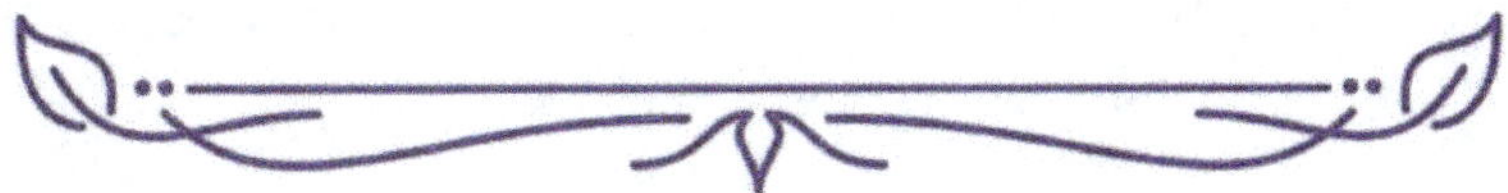

This scrub is perfect for a relaxing night in. The exfoliating power of African black soap and organic sugar helps to remove dead skin cells, while the moisturizing shea butter and coconut oil leave your skin feeling soft and smooth. The soothing aroma of chamomile essential oil will help you relax and unwind before bed.

Ingredients:

- ½ cup organic unrefined shea butter, whipped
- 3 tablespoons organic virgin coconut oil
- 1 teaspoon Roman chamomile essential oil
- ¼ cup liquid or softened African black soap
- ½ cup organic sugar

Instructions:

1. In a bowl, combine the shea butter, coconut oil, and chamomile essential oil.
2. Mix until well combined.
3. Add the African black soap and sugar and mix until a thick paste forms.
4. Apply the scrub to your damp skin in a gentle, circular motion.
5. Leave the scrub on for 10-15 minutes, then rinse it off with warm water.

Tips:

- You can store this scrub in an airtight container in the refrigerator for up to 2 weeks.

- If you have sensitive skin, you may want to start with a smaller amount of the scrub and gradually increase the amount as your skin gets used to it.

- Avoid using this scrub on open wounds or irritated skin.

Enjoy your relaxing night in!

NOURISHING

FACIAL WIPES

These DIY facial wipes are so simple and affordable to make, you'll wonder how you ever lived without them! They're perfect for removing makeup, dirt, and oil from your face, and they're gentle enough for everyday use.

Ingredients:

- 12-15 paper towel sheets, cut in half
- 2 cups distilled water
- 3 tablespoons organic virgin coconut oil
- ½ cup witch hazel
- 1 tablespoon organic liquid or softened African black soap*
- 1 teaspoon essential oil of choice (optional)

Instructions:

1. Cut the paper towels in half and then fold them into small squares.
2. Stack the paper towels in a large, clean, wide-mouth glass jar.
3. In a separate bowl, combine the distilled water, witch hazel, coconut oil, essential oil, and African black soap. Stir vigorously until the water and oil are well mixed.
4. Immediately pour the cleansing solution into the glass jar, covering the paper towels.
5. Secure the lid on the jar and shake to make sure all of the paper towels are coated with the cleansing solution.

To use:

1. Remove a paper towel square from the jar.

2. Use the paper towel to gently wash your face and remove makeup and dirt.

3. Wipe your face with a clean washcloth.

4. These wipes are great at removing eye makeup, but be careful not to get any of the cleansing solution in your eyes.

Storage:

Keep the lid closed tightly on the jar. The cleansing solution should be good for up to four weeks.

Tips:

- You can use any essential oil that you like. Some popular choices for facial wipes include lavender, chamomile, and rose.

- If you have sensitive skin, you may want to use a gentler essential oil, such as lavender or chamomile.

- You can also add a few drops of aloe vera juice to the cleansing solution for extra hydration.

- Store the wipes in the refrigerator for a refreshingly cool experience.

I hope you enjoy making and using these DIY facial wipes!

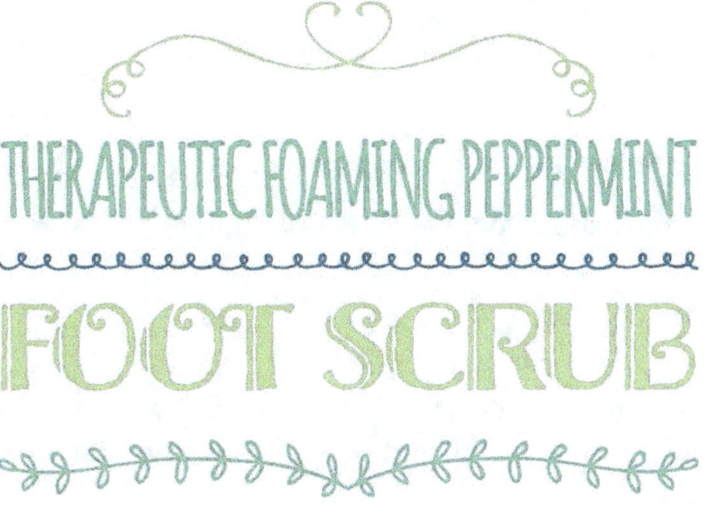
THERAPEUTIC FOAMING PEPPERMINT
FOOT SCRUB

This easy foot scrub is perfect for soothing tired, dry feet. The Epsom salt and Himalayan salt help to exfoliate the skin, while the African black soap, sweet almond oil, and peppermint essential oil leave your feet feeling tingly and fresh.

Ingredients:

- 1 cup Epsom salt
- 2 tablespoons organic pink Himalayan salt
- 3 tablespoons organic liquid or softened African black soap
- 4 tablespoons sweet almond oil
- 1 tablespoon peppermint essential oil

Instructions:

1. In a medium bowl, combine the African black soap, sweet almond oil, and peppermint essential oil.
2. Stir in the Epsom salt and Himalayan salt until well combined.
3. Transfer the scrub to an airtight container.

To use:

1. Apply the scrub to your feet and massage in a circular motion.
2. Leave the scrub on for 5-10 minutes, then rinse it off with warm water.

3. Pat your feet dry and apply a moisturizer.

Tips:

- You can store the scrub in an airtight container in the refrigerator for up to 2 weeks.

- If you have sensitive skin, you may want to start with a smaller amount of the scrub and gradually increase the amount as your skin gets used to it.

- Avoid using the scrub on open wounds or irritated skin.

Enjoy your refreshed, tingly feet!

AFRICAN BLACK SOAP FOAMING FACIAL WASH

Why spend a lot of money on department store facial washes when you can make this one at home for just a few dollars using all-natural ingredients?

Ingredients:

- ¼ cup organic liquid or softened African black soap
- ¾ cup brewed organic chamomile tea
- ½ teaspoon organic aloe vera gel
- ½ teaspoon organic unrefined whipped shea butter
- 5-6 drops of lavender essential oil (optional)

Instructions:

1. In a clean jar, combine the African black soap, chamomile tea, aloe vera gel, and shea butter.
2. Add the essential oil, if using.
3. Stir until well combined.
4. Transfer the face wash to a pump bottle.

To use:

1. Pump 2-3 times into your palm.
2. Apply the face wash to your face and neck.
3. Massage in a circular motion for 1 minute.
4. Rinse thoroughly with warm water.

This face wash is gentle enough for daily use and can help to cleanse, exfoliate, and moisturize your skin. The chamomile tea is soothing and calming, while the lavender essential oil is relaxing and refreshing.

Enjoy your homemade face wash!

Here are some additional tips:

- You can use any type of essential oil that you like. Some other popular choices for face washes include tea tree oil, rose oil, and geranium oil.

- If you have sensitive skin, you may want to start with a smaller amount of essential oil and gradually increase the amount as your skin gets used to it.

- You can store the face wash in a cool, dark place for up to 2 weeks.

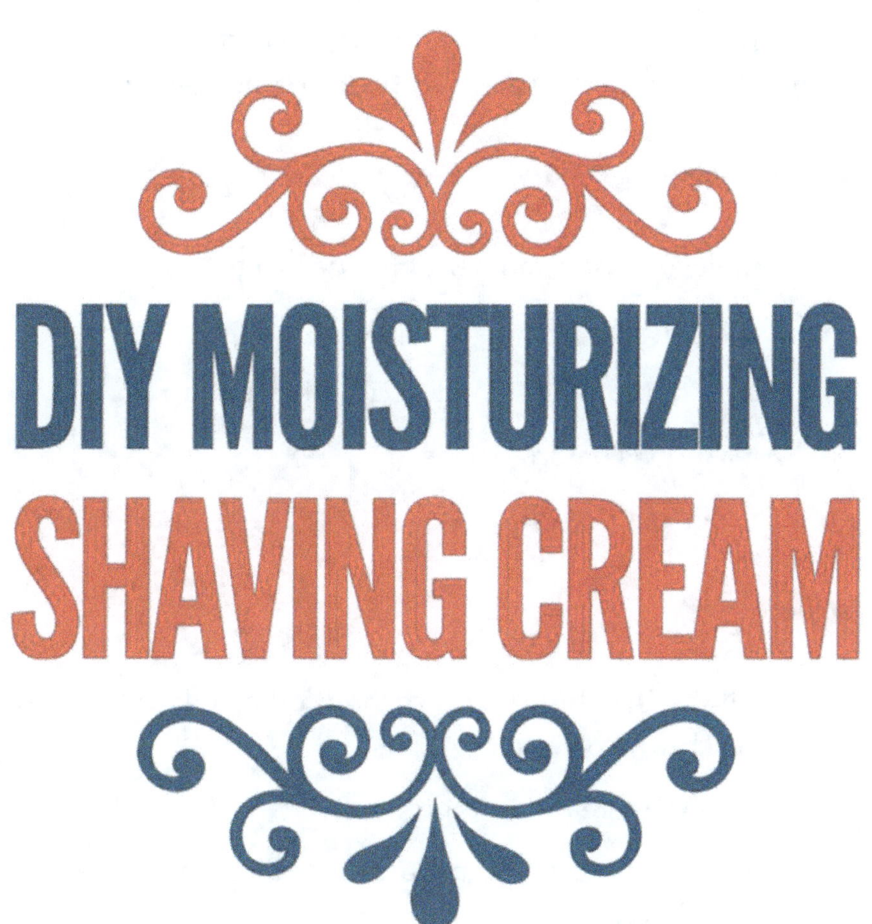

DIY MOISTURIZING
SHAVING CREAM

This DIY whipped shaving cream recipe is a great way to get a close, comfortable shave without using harsh chemicals or artificial ingredients. The shea butter and coconut oil will moisturize your skin, while the baking soda and African black soap will help to exfoliate and prevent razor bumps. The tea tree oil is an added bonus, as it has antibacterial and anti-inflammatory properties that can help to soothe any irritation.

Ingredients:

- 2 tablespoons organic unrefined shea butter
- ⅓ cup organic virgin coconut oil
- ¼ cup liquid or softened African black soap
- 2 teaspoons baking soda
- 5 drops tea tree oil

Instructions:

1. Melt the shea butter and coconut oil in a double boiler or in the microwave.
2. Stir in the remaining ingredients.
3. Pour the mixture into a glass jar and refrigerate for at least 30 minutes.
4. Once the mixture is cool, whip it with a hand mixer until it is light and fluffy.
5. Store the shaving cream in an airtight container in the refrigerator. It will last for up to 1-2 months.

Tips:

- For the best shave, start with a clean, sharp razor.

- Apply a thin layer of shaving cream to your skin.

- Rinse the razor blades as needed while shaving.

- Pat your skin dry with a clean towel after shaving.

This shaving cream is perfect for all skin types, including sensitive skin. It is also a great option for people who are looking for a natural and cruelty-free shaving cream.

I hope you enjoy this recipe!

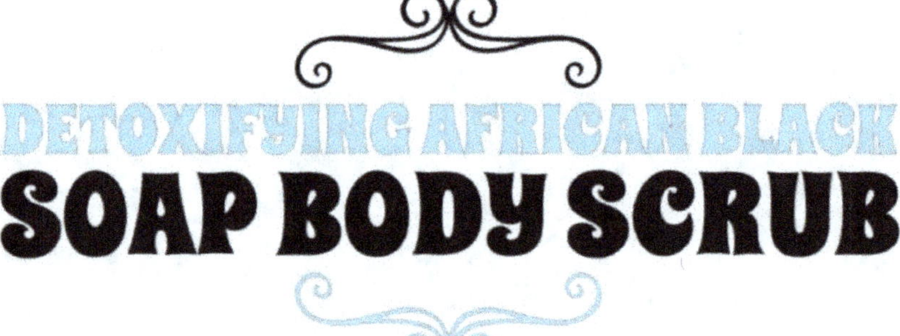DETOXIFYING AFRICAN BLACK
SOAP BODY SCRUB

This DIY detoxifying and moisturizing scrub is a great way to exfoliate your skin and remove dead skin cells. The shea butter and jojoba oil moisturize your skin, while the Himalayan salt and African black soap exfoliate and detoxify your skin. The juniper and black pepper essential oils add a refreshing scent and have antibacterial properties.

Ingredients:

- ¼ cup organic unrefined shea butter
- ¼ cup organic liquid or softened African black soap
- 1 cup fine organic pink Himalayan salt
- 30 drops juniper essential oil
- 5 drops black pepper essential oil
- 15 drops jojoba oil

Instructions:

1. Mix all the ingredients in a medium-sized bowl.
2. Store in an airtight glass jar.
3. Massage the scrub onto your skin gently, starting from your feet and working upwards.
4. If you have sensitive skin, avoid using this scrub on your face.
5. Rinse the remains of the scrub off with warm water.

Tips:

- You can adjust the amount of essential oils to your liking.

- If you don't have jojoba oil, you can substitute another carrier oil, such as almond oil or coconut oil.

- This scrub can be stored in an airtight container in the refrigerator for up to 2 weeks.

Make this DIY detoxifying and moisturizing scrub today and enjoy soft, smooth, and detoxified skin!

BUBBLING FOOT
SCRUB &
SOAK
FOR CALLUSES

This DIY African black soap and salt scrub is a natural and effective way to exfoliate and moisturize your feet, leaving them feeling soft, smooth, and refreshed. The Epsom salt and sea salt help to remove dead skin cells, while the African black soap cleanses and detoxifies your feet. The olive oil moisturizes your feet and helps to prevent further dryness. The peppermint essential oil is optional, but it adds a refreshing scent and has antibacterial properties.

Ingredients:

- 3 tablespoons organic liquid or softened African black soap
- 2 cups Epsom salt
- ½ cup organic sea salt
- 1 tablespoon organic olive oil
- 2-3 drops peppermint essential oil (optional)

Instructions:

1. Combine the Epsom salt, sea salt, African black soap, and olive oil in a large bowl. Stir well until combined.
2. Store the scrub in an airtight glass jar.

To use as a scrub:

1. Add ½ cup of the scrub to warm water.
2. Soak your feet for 15 minutes.

3. Use a loofah or pumice stone to gently slough off dead skin cells.

To use as a soak:

1. Add 1 cup of the scrub to a warm bath.

2. Soak your feet for 20-30 minutes.

3. For extra moisturizing, apply shea butter to your feet and then put on cotton socks.

Tips:

- You can adjust the amount of peppermint essential oil to your liking.

- If you don't have peppermint essential oil, you can substitute another essential oil, such as lavender or eucalyptus.

- This scrub can be stored in an airtight container in the refrigerator for up to 2 weeks.

Soothing eczema

BATH SOAK

Eczema is a common skin condition that causes redness, itching, and inflammation. It can be triggered by a variety of factors, including stress, allergies, and dry skin. This DIY bath soak is a gentle and effective way to soothe eczema and relieve symptoms.

Ingredients:

- 1 tablespoon organic liquid or softened African black soap
- 1 cup Epsom salts
- ¼ cup organic apple cider vinegar
- 1 cup baking soda
- ¼ teaspoon lemon essential oil
- ¼ teaspoon lavender essential oil

Instructions:

1. Combine the baking soda and Epsom salts in a bowl. Stir to blend.
2. Pour ¼ cup of the mixture into the bathtub while the water is running.
3. Add the apple cider vinegar, African black soap, and essential oils to the bath water and stir to combine.
4. Soak in the bath for 20-30 minutes.

Tips:

- The water should be warm, but not too hot.

- You can adjust the amount of essential oils to your liking.

- If you don't have lemon or lavender essential oils, you can substitute other essential oils that are soothing for eczema, such as chamomile or rose.

- This bath soak can be used as often as needed.

Warning:

- Do not take hot baths or salt baths if you have high blood pressure, heart problems, or are a diabetic.

Enjoy your soothing and relaxing bath soak!

CONCLUSION

In this guide, you have learned about all the amazing health benefits of African black soap. You also found out how to care for different skin types and utilize African black soap to address your skin care needs. However, it is important to use it safely. Here are a few safety guidelines to keep in mind:

- Do not ingest African black soap. It is not meant to be eaten and can cause stomach upset or other health problems.

- If you get African black soap in your eyes, rinse them immediately and thoroughly with water. Do not rub your eyes.

- African black soap can be drying to the skin, so it is important to moisturize after using it.

- If you have sensitive skin, you may want to patch test African black soap on a small area of your skin before using it all over.

- If you experience any irritation or allergic reaction after using African black soap, discontinue use and consult a doctor.

Here are some additional tips for using African black soap safely:

- Start with a small amount of soap and gradually increase the amount as needed.

- Apply the soap to wet skin and massage it in gently.

- Rinse the soap off thoroughly with warm water.

- Use African black soap as often as needed but avoid using it every day if you have sensitive skin.

If you have a negative reaction to African black soap, stop using it and consult your doctor or dermatologist.

Now that you know all about the wonderful health benefits of this all-natural soap, you can start incorporating it into your daily skin routine. The skin care recipes in this book are highly customizable and versatile, so you can adjust them to fit your skin type and lifestyle. If you don't have a certain ingredient available, you can simply substitute it! Just make sure to use a carrier oil and exfoliant that is all natural and appropriate for your skin type.

You can find organic raw unrefined African black soap bars, organic liquid African black soap, and organic whipped unrefined shea butter on our website: www.frafrasnaturals.com. We carry a variety of liquid African black soap and whipped unrefined shea butters mixed with essential oils.

FAQ ABOUT FRA FRA'S NATURALS

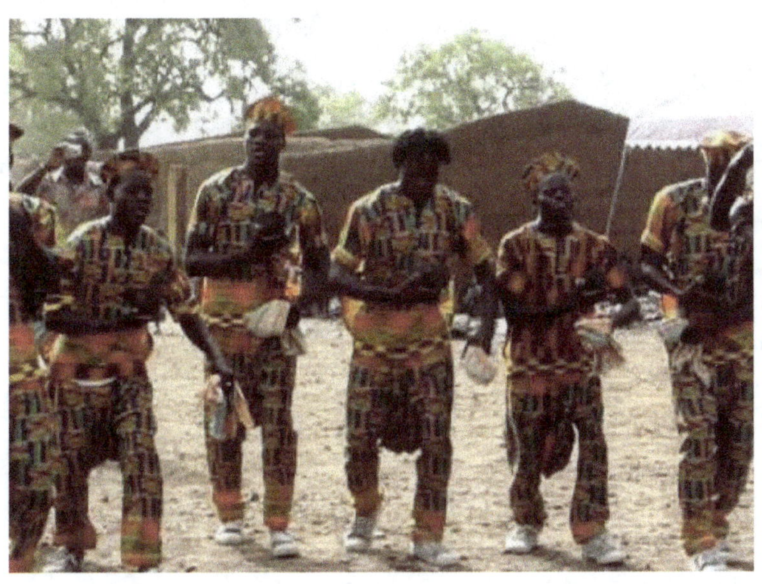

Question: Where does the name Fra Fra (pronounced fray fray) come from?

Answer: The name Fra Fra comes from my husband's nickname, which he got when he was younger. People used to call him Fra Fra because it sounded like his last name, Frazier. I recently found out that there is a tribe in Northern Ghana called the Fra Fra tribe, and they are the primary source of black soap and shea butter. When I started selling black soap and shea butter, I knew that I had to name my business Fra Fra's. It felt like kismet!

Question: Who is the Fra Fra tribe?

Answer: The Fra Fra tribe is a subset of the Gur people living in northern Ghana. The name Fra Fra comes from the tribe's traditional greeting, "Ya Fara-Fara?", which means "How is your suffering (work)?". They are a sedentary agricultural tribe that grows all kinds of staples such as beans, maize, rice, and yams. There are approximately 300,000 Fra Fra speakers.

Question: I don't see the essential oil blend I need. Do you take requests?

Answer: Yes, we do! Please contact us if you would like for us to source an essential oil combination for you. We have a wide variety of essential oils available, and we can customize a blend to meet your specific needs.

Question: Are you on social media?

Answer: Yes! Please follow us for exclusive sales and discounts:

 @frafrasnaturals

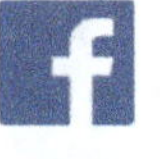 Fra Fras Naturals Shea Butter and black soap

 @frafrasnaturals

 Frafrasnaturals